DEERHURST CONSUM

GW00976537

THE
MEDICINE BOOK

DEERHURST PUBLICATIONS

CONTENTS

Published by
Deerhurst Publications
Ashburton House
26 Dyke Drive
Orpington
Kent
BR5 4LZ

© Deerhurst Publications 1991

ISBN 1 8735 19 109

Typeset, printed and bound by
BPCC-AUP Aberdeen Ltd

INTRODUCTION—ABOUT THIS BOOK

Have you ever been to the chemist, for say some cough medicine, only to be confronted by two shelves full of bottles and not known which one to pick. This book has been written to hopefully save you from this problem by listing out the most popular medicines available to treat many common ailments and conditions.

This book however is *NOT* a guide to self prescription, nor is it a home doctor. It is simply a guide to what is available in your chemist shop or from your doctor (G.P.). We hope it will be useful for families and individuals who want to know about the range of medicines and treatments available for a particular condition or problem.

We have specifically omitted the more serious diseases since these should always be treated by a doctor and their advice should be taken. In all cases the advice of a pharmacist or doctor should be sought before medication is commenced and this is especially true for a patient who is already taking other medicines.

Finally use this book in conjunction with your doctor and pharmacist. If you have a bad cough for instance, look up the entry on cough's to see which of the medicines listed might suit you best. Then speak to your pharmacist and ask for their advice. See if this really is the best medicine for you and if it is not, use the book with your pharmacist's help to see what really would be best suited for your needs. Alternatively if your doctor has prescribed a drug which doesn't seem to work for you, use the book to see which alternative's are available and then discuss with him or her whether a change of drug might be a good idea.

In all, use this book to help you choose and use the drugs best suited to you and remember if in doubt, a Pharmacist is always well qualified to give you the best advice concerning your medication.

HOW TO USE THIS BOOK

The entries in this book are laid out in alphabetical order. So if you wish to look up the medicines available for any particular ailment then simply turn to that entry.

Once you have turned to a page you will see that there is a short description of the condition at the top. Here will be noted any important points or comments that might need to be made. This is followed by two lists. One concerning all the drugs which are available from the chemist and a second on those available from the doctor. Always remember that the doctor may prescribe drugs which are also available without prescription from the chemist.

Each list is itself divided into three columns. The first column lists the medicines available. The medicines in bold are the main drug type, and these are followed by the different varieties of this drug that are available. The second column contains information that might be relevant to either a particular drug or a group of drugs in general. The final column lists some of the more common side effects that might occur. It is important to note though that these are only POSSIBLE side effects and there is no suggestion that any or all of these reactions will necessarily take place.

It is important to note that the Chemist's and Doctors medicines lists are not mutually exclusive and as mentioned above drugs may occur on both lists.

ACNE

A skin condition commonly occurring in teenagers although it can appear at any age under certain conditions. It affects mainly face, neck, back and chest. Caused by excessive oil production by the skin and results in blackheads, inflamed spots and pustules (whiteheads). Mild acne can be treated by frequent washing together with a topical (skin) preparation to keep the skin clean and oil free. Severe acne can be treated by prescription drugs and creams from your doctor. Both forms require regular and long term treatment.

DRUGS FROM CHEMIST

Drug	Information	Possible Side Effects
Salicylic acid preparations —Clearasil —OxyClean	These remove dead skin cells which block pores and allow bacteria to cause infection.	Over use can lead to skin irritation.
Benzoyl peroxide —Acetoxyl —Acnegel —Benoxyl —Oxy 5/10 —Panoxy —Quinoderm —Ultra Clearasil	Has an antibacterial effect. Reduces inflammation caused by infection and removes top layer of skin to unblock pores.	Over use causes skin irritation, dry skin and peeling. Do not use for longer than six weeks.
Phenoxypropanol —Biactol —Phytocil	Has an antibacterial effect. Reduces inflammation caused by bacteria.	Over use can lead to skin irritation.

DRUGS FROM DOCTOR

Drug	Information	Possible Side Effects
Oral antibiotics —Co-trimoxazole —Minocycline —Oxytetracycline	For moderate to severe acne; these are taken on long-term basis to kill bacteria and cure inflammation.	Nausea, diarrhoea, vaginal thrush. Rashes.
Isotretinoin	For very severe acne; this is very effective.	Dry, cracked lips, dry eyes, nosebleeds and headaches.
Dalacin T	Topical antibiotic lotion which reduces bacterial infection and inflammation.	Skin rash/irritation.

CONSULT YOUR DOCTOR OR PHARMACIST BEFORE TAKING MEDICATION

ANAEMIA

Anaemia is a disorder of the red blood cells which can cause tiredness, breathlessness and dizziness. Usually due to a deficiency of iron in the diet. The main treatment recommended for mild deficiency is to increase intake of foods containing iron such as liver.

DRUGS FROM CHEMIST

Drug	Information	Possible Side Effects
Iron preparations, Vitamin B12 preparations	These contain too little of the required amount to be effective— always seek a doctor's advice.	Not significant unless taken in large amounts.

DRUGS FROM DOCTOR

Drug	Information	Possible Side Effects
Iron tablets —Ferrous compounds	For iron deficiencies, replace lost stores.	Nausea, constipation, diarrhoea, (dark faeces).
Iron injections e.g. Iron Dectran	—ditto—	Nausea, vomiting, flushing.
Folic Acid Tablets	Rapid recovery.	No significant SE.
Vitamin B12 tablets and injections (Cyanocobalamin).	Maintenance doses may be required.	No significant SE.

ANTIBACTERIALS

These drugs were the first to be used against bacteria. Today, Antibiotics are used more often, but in some cases such as urinary infections, the antibacterials may be considered more effective. Always complete a course of treatment even if your symptoms clear up. Antibacterials, like some antibiotics, may cause allergic reactions in the patient. Also nausea and diarrhoea.

DRUGS FROM DOCTOR

Drug	Information	Possible Side Effects
Sulphonamides —Co-trimoxazole (Septrin or Septrin Forte a stronger version)	Used for urinary tract infections and for some ear infections. A general purpose antibacterial.	See introduction above.
Urinary Drugs —Nalidixic Acid —Nitrofurantoin	Both these drugs used as urinary antiseptics.	
Other Drugs —Chloramphenicol	Mainly for eye use. Very potent and only used orally for serious conditions due to possible side effects.	
—Dapsone	Mainly for skin use.	
—Metronidazole	For general infections including genital infections.	Must avoid alcohol.
—Trimethoprim	With Sulpha-methoxazole for bladder infections/bronchitis and intestinal problems. Also used on its own in certain infections.	

ANTIBIOTICS

This is a class of drugs which are used to control bacterial and certain fungal infections. Bacteria live harmlessly all around us, but become harmful when they enter body areas they do not normally exist in. It can then be said that the bacteria have infected that area of the body. Such infections can be spread by insects, food, water, touch and sexual contact.

The bacteria produce poisons which may cause many different symptoms in the infected person. These symptoms can differ depending on where the bacteria are in the body. Swelling may occur with a skin infection while fever, sickness and diarrhoea can be seen where the bacteria have been consumed in contaminated food or water.

To fight bacteria we can use antibiotics. These fight the infection by either killing the bacteria outright or stopping their reproduction. There are several groups of antibiotics which all have slightly different properties. Some may work against many common bacteria and are said to have a broad spectrum. Others may however be more specific and are said to have a narrow spectrum. Some antibiotics are more suitable in severe infections or certain situations. The GP will choose an antibiotic which he or she thinks will be most effective in a particular situation. Very few antibiotics can be bought over the counter. This is because if too many antibiotics are taken needlessly, the bacteria can build up a resistance to them.

If rashes occur with any penicillin drug or tetracycline then inform GP at once or ask a Pharmacist for advice.

DRUGS FROM CHEMIST

Drug	Information	Possible Side Effects
Brolene	Available as eye drops/Eye ointment for slight conjunctivitis.	Possible eye irritation.

ANTIBIOTICS *(continued)*

DRUGS FROM DOCTOR

Drug	Information	Possible Side Effects
Aminoglycosides —Gentamicin —Neomycin —Netilmicin —Streptomycin —Tobramycin	Useful for Ear, nose and throat, skin, kidney and stomach/intestinal infections. Usually only given by injection in hospitals. Broad spectrum.	Possible skin rashes and kidney problems.
Cephalosporins —Cefaclor —Cephalothin —Cefoxitin —Cephalexin —Cephazolin	Can be given by mouth or injection. May be used as an alternative when penicillins do not work. Broad spectrum.	May cause allergic reactions similar to penicillin.
Macrolides —Erythromycin	Broad spectrum.	Very occasionally impairs liver function
Penicillins —Amoxycillin —Ampicillin —Benzylpenicillin —Cloxacillin —Penicillin V	The first antibiotics discovered and still used today. However many bacteria have built up a resistance to the drug.	May cause allergic reactions such as sickness, nausea and rashes.
Tetracyclines —Doxycycline —Oxytetracycline —Tetracycline	These drugs have a very broad spectrum. However due to the bacteria's ability to develop resistance they are of less use than they used to be.	Should not be taken with milk or iron tablets as they may reduce the drugs efficiency. Also because of the need to maintain high blood levels, drug may cause diarrhoea. May cause discolouring in developing teeth. Do not use in children under 12 years of age or pregnant women.
Augmentin	Contains amoxycillin with clavulanic acid. This makes the antibiotic more effective against certain infections.	Nausea, diarrhoea and rashes.

CONSULT YOUR DOCTOR OR PHARMACIST BEFORE TAKING MEDICATION

ANTIHISTAMINES

Antihistamines are drugs that are able to reduce the amount of histamine in the body. Histamines are chemicals which undertake a number of roles. They are released when the body is subjected to an allergic reaction. Other functions include widening and closing of the body's blood vessels, contraction of the gastrointestinal tract and respiratory muscles. Also the release of digestive juices in the stomach.

Antihistamines are able to counteract these effects. They are used particularly in hay fever and general allergic reactions. They are able to reduce swelling and itching. They work best if used before an allergic reaction takes place.

DRUGS FROM CHEMIST (may also be prescribed by your doctor

Drug	Information	Possible Side Effects
Azatadine —Optimine	These drugs are used to deal with allergic reactions such as hay fever and Urticaria (acute or chronic allergic skin reaction).	Drowsiness can be a major side effect when using antihistamines. Other side effects include headaches, dry mouth, blurred vision and constipation.
Brompheniramine —Dimotane		
Chlorpheniramine —Piriton		
Clemastine —Aller-eze	Most of these antihistamines can be given as tablets, syrups and elixirs. Sometimes given by injection.	Avoid alcohol.
Promethazine —Phenergan		Some modern antihistamines cause less drowsiness.
Terfenadine —Triludan	A non sedative antihistamine.	
Astemizole —Hismanal —Pollon-eze	As Terfenadine.	

DRUGS FROM DOCTOR

Drug	Information	Possible Side Effects
Acrivastine —Semprex	These are predominantly non-sedative antihistamines.	These do not cause drowsiness.
Cetirizine —Zirtex		
Trimeprazine —Vallergan	This is a sedative antihistamine.	

Anxiety or nerves/nervous tension can be brought about by a whole variety of causes. Stress however is most common. This can be stress caused by work pressures, family problems, bereavement or money problems. The end result is often the same. A range of physical feelings can be encountered which may include edginess, irritability, dry mouth, tense muscles, pains in the chest and severe panic attacks, dizziness and sweating.

These feelings themselves can be just a nuisance or spread to ruin the quality of your whole life. Everyone encounters anxiety at some time in their life. However if the anxiety rises to such a point that they can't cope with it any more, many may turn to pills to help them cope. It should be said however, especially considering the many side effects which may occur as a result of tranquilizers, that counselling and self help may be a better bet than drugs. Certainly it seems ill advised to take tranquilizers on a very long term basis.

DRUGS FROM CHEMIST

None are available over the counter. Relaxation exercises can be beneficial in controlling symptoms. Counselling can also help discover cause of anxiety. Herbal remedies and homoeopathy are also available but their usefulness has still not been proven.

DRUGS FROM DOCTOR

Drug	Information	Possible Side Effects
Tranquillizers (Benzodiazepines). —Alprazolam; —Diazepam; —Lorazepam.	Relieve for 6-weeks. Act on brain to calm patient, have different duration of action. Lorazepam both acts quicker and leaves the body quicker than Diazepam. However the body develops a tolerance to Lorazepam quicker and so a greater dose is needed to achieve the same result.	Drowsiness, lethargy, lack of concentration and memory. Possible addiction after 6-months. Carries the increased risk of wiithdrawal symptoms.
Beta blockers —Propranolol —Oxprenolol	Reduce physical symptoms of anxiety e.g. palpitations.	Tiredness, cold hands and feet. Non-addictive. Do not take if asthmatic.

CONSULT YOUR DOCTOR OR PHARMACIST BEFORE TAKING MEDICATION

ARTHRITIS—RHEUMATOID

This is a chronic (slow on-setting) inflammation of the joints causing deformity and disability of the body. There will be swelling and stiffness of the affected joints. Often in the hands and feet first. Over a period of time the disease can spread causing overall fatigue, loss of appetite and weight loss. The symptoms can be very severe at times and then reduce at other times.

DRUGS FROM CHEMIST

Drug	Information	Possible Side Effects
Paracetamol	This is a useful short term pain killer. Unlike asprin it does not interfere with other drugs. Do NOT however self medicate, but always consult your doctor.	Can cause liver damage in over dose.

The doctor should be consulted over this condition. If your doctor has already given you drugs for arthritis but you still feel pain then go back to him. DO NOT take additional painkillers without consulting a GP or a pharmacist as these may cause you to exceed the daily limit of your medicine.

DRUGS FROM DOCTOR

Drug	Information	Possible Side Effects
NSAID's —Ibuprofen; —Aspirin; —Ketoprofen; —Indomethacin.	These reduce inflammation and also help the pain of joints. See Pain.	Stomach discomfort, nausea and stomach bleeding. Aggravates stomach ulcers—Should not be taken by people to asprin.
Antirheumatic drugs —Chloroquine; —Penicillamine; —Sodium aurothiomalate. (Gold).	Reduce inflammation and pain, but take several months to work effectively.	Skin rashes, nausea. 'Gold Cards' must be carried in case of sudden reaction. Regular urine and blood checks are important.
Steroids e.g. Prednisolone	Reduce inflammation while treatment lasts. Side effects would be reduced by use of steroid injections rather than tablets.	If used only for a short time, side effects are rare. Do not stop taking these suddenly.

ATHLETES FOOT

This condition is also called 'tinea pedis' and is caused by a fungal infection. It can either appear as a red, sore flaky area between the toes or perhaps small blisters which cause peeling of the skin. It is caused by the moist conditions between the toes and sufferers should keep their feet as clean and dry as possible. Apply cream to the area and dust socks and shoes thoroughly with powder daily. Do not swim or walk barefoot in public areas until the infection is cleared up and ensure towels are kept separate from the family.

DRUGS FROM CHEMIST (may also be available from the doctor

Drug	Information	Possible Side Effects
Tolnaftate 1% preps —Mycil —Tineaderm —Tineafax —Timoped	These contain an antifungal agent which should be used daily for at least two weeks to clear up the infection.	Rare sensitivity.
Zinc Undecanoate —Mycota	Also an antifungal agent and requires continual use for about two to three weeks.	None significant.
Salicylic acid preps —Phytocil	Available as a cream applied two or three times daily.	Hypersensitivity.
Clotrimazole —Canesten	An antifungal cream. Apply two or three times daily.	Rare skin irritation.

DRUGS FROM DOCTOR

Drug	Information	Possible Side Effects
Miconazole —Daktarin **Econazole** —Pevaryl	Use creams 2-3 times a day for up to 4 weeks. Powder should not be applied to broken skin. Treatment should be continued for 2 weeks after cure. Always ensure that the area around infected skin is sufficiently treated.	Skin irritation

There are a variety of strong antifungal preparations which your doctor may prescribe. Most infections however will clear up with good hygeine and regular use of products from the chemist shop.

CONSULT YOUR DOCTOR OR PHARMACIST BEFORE TAKING MEDICATION

BACK PAIN (Ache)

Persistant back pain may need other treatment apart from usual painkillers. Your doctor should be consulted if it lasts for several days.

DRUGS FROM CHEMIST

There are a number of painkillers of different strengths available. See section on Pain.

DRUGS FROM DOCTOR

Drug	Information	Possible Side Effects
Muscle relaxants: —Diazepam; —Chlormezanone.	Used when pain is due to muscle spasm.	Drowsiness, blurred vision in high doses.
Narcotic analgesics: —Dihydrocodeine; —Buprenorphine.	Strong pain relievers.	Constipation. Addictive in long term. Nausea, drowsiness
NSAID's: —Ibuprofen; —Indomethacin.	Reduce pain by reducing swelling and inflammation.	Indigestion, take with food.
Simple analgesics: —Aspirin; —Paracetamol.	Reduce inflammation and relieve pain. No antiinflammatory effect.	Few. Aspirin can cause stomach upset. Do **not** give to UNDER-12's.

CANDIDA (See Fungal Infections)

Most children will catch some form of illness during their early years. Mostly these are coughs, colds and sneezes, but it can be worrying if they develop one of the more serious childhood ailments. These diseases almost always need to be checked out by a doctor, but surprisingly there is little that can be done for most of the common viral complaints and it is these that make up most of the childhood illnesses.

Many doctors consider it is better if the child is immunised to prevent them catching the disease in the first place. However some of these vaccines themselves create a deal of controversy over their use and any possible side effects they might cause (Discuss this with your doctor if in doubt). Below is a selection of common childhood complaints. If in doubt always consult the doctor. Do not be surprised however if he or she suggests a 'wait and see' policy. Many are reluctant to over prescribe antibiotics in case a resistance builds up and so may prefer to see if the condition clears up on its own first.

Children's Viral infections include:

Measles	These are all viral diseases and antibiotics have little
Mumps	effect except to stop secondary infections.
Chicken Pox	
Whooping Cough	Whooping cough, German measles and Mumps all have
Scarlet Fever	Vaccines, available.
German Measles	

DRUGS FROM CHEMIST

Drug	Information	Possible Side Effects
Paracetamol —Panadol —Calpol.	Used to treat pain and fever. Comes in junior form for children and a variety of trade names.	Use only in accordance with instructions on the bottle.

Cont...

CONSULT YOUR DOCTOR OR PHARMACIST BEFORE TAKING MEDICATION

CHILDRENS AILMENTS *(continued)*

DRUGS FROM DOCTOR

Drug	Information	Possible Side Effects
Antibiotics: —Amoxycillin; —Erythromycin.	These kill bacteria and prevent viral infections leading to secondary diseases and bacteria infections. See Antibiotics.	Occasional mild diarrhoea.
Anti-worm preps. —Mebendazole; —Piperazine.	These rid the body of small worms picked up from pets or dirt/sand. Usually given as a one or two dose powder. Follow instructions exactly and treat the whole family	

CHICKEN POX (See Childrens Ailments)

COLDS

These are viral infections for which there is no real curative treatment. Usually any drugs used will only make the symptoms more bearable. Symptoms include runny or congested noses. Headache, raised temperature and general feeling of illhealth. Antibiotics may be used with care to prevent secondary infections.

DRUGS FROM CHEMIST

Drug	Information	Possible Side Effects
Pain Killers (analgesics): —see PAIN	Help to lower patient's temperature and ease headaches and general pain. Paracetamol syrups are available for children.	See PAIN. Do not give aspirin to children under 12 years.
Decongestants: —Actifed —Congesteze —Dimotane —Dimotapp —Galpseud —Sudafed —Triogesic	These dry up nasal secretions and reduce swelling.	Should not be used on patients with high blood pressure or heart disease. May also cause drowsiness. Avoid alcohol. Should not be taken when pregnant.
Nose drops Local decongestant —Ephedrine —Saline nose drops —Sinex. —Otrivine	As above.	These should be used with care. They may damage the nasal membranes and cause more congestion in the long run.
Combination symptom Relievers Night Nurse Contact 400 Sudafed Co and others	These are combination treatments containing paracetamol, a decongestant and antihistamine in different combinations.	Take care not to overdose on the Paracetamol.

DRUGS FROM DOCTOR

Drug	Information	Possible Side Effects
Antibiotics: see ANTIBIOTICS	Treat bacterial infections.	Nausea and usual side effects.

CONSULT YOUR DOCTOR OR PHARMACIST BEFORE TAKING MEDICATION

COLD SORES (Herpes simplex)

Cold Sores are caused by a virus carried by many of the population. It is seen as a painful sore around the lips. These attacks can occur at various times and start with a stinging, itching sensation around the infected area.

DRUGS FROM CHEMIST

Drug	Information	Possible Side Effects
Liquids/lotions —Blisteze	These liquids supposedly 'dry-up' the Cold Sores, but are of only limited use.	Stinging on use.

DRUGS FROM DOCTOR

Drug	Information	Possible Side Effects
Antiviral Creams —Acyclovir (Zovirax)	Used as a Cream as quickly as possible when the first signs of the Cold Sore show themselves. Once the sore is developed then the cream will have little effect. Get some from your Doctor and store in the fridge until needed.	Not to be used in pregnancy. Rashes.

14

CONSTIPATION

This is a condition where a person passes fewer and harder motions (or stools) than is normal for them. One of the common causes is lack of roughage in a person's diet and an increase in food containing fibre may often improve the problem. Laxatives should not be used on a continual basis. If they are required for a long period then a visit to the doctor might be needed to get some advice on diet.

DRUGS FROM CHEMIST

Drug	Information	Possible Side Effects
Osmotic Laxatives: —Lactulose —Duphalac Milk of Magnesia Epsom/liver salts Andrews Eno's 'Fruit Salts' Citric Acid Tartaric Acid	They increase the water content of the bowel motion. May cause salt and water retention.	Slight possibility of flatulence or dehydration. Long term use may cause blood chemical imbalances. Do not take the so called "health salts" with congestive heart disease.
Stimulant Laxatives: —Bisacodyl —Dulcolax —Toilex —Perilax	Stimulates the bowel muscle. Takes about 12 hours to have effect.	If taken in excess cause diarrhoea or stomach cramps. Doses may vary depending on the person.
Cascara Castor Oil Fig Senna —Senokot	Works quicker than most other stimulate laxatives since it works on the small intestine. About 3 hours.	May cause bowel irritation. Avoid if alternatives are available.
Phenolphthalein —Ex-lax —Alophen —Brooklax —Nylax		May cause urine to colour pink or allergic skin reactions.

Cont...

CONSTIPATION *(continued)*

DRUGS FROM CHEMIST

Drug	Information	Possible Side Effects
Lubricant Laxatives:	Soften and lubricate motions. Can take up to 48 hours to have effect. Prevent straining.	
Mineral Oils —Liquid Paraffin	Avoid if possible.	May effect Vitamin A and D absorption.
Dioctyl Sodium Sulphocuccinate —Docusate Sodium —Normax —Dulcodos	Act as a sort of wetting agent which softens the motions	
Bulking agents: —Celevac —Fybogel —Regulan —Normacol	Increase bulk of bowl contents. Take about 12-24 hours to have effect. Take with plenty of water.	Do not take at bedtime.
Suppositories —Bisacodyl —Glycerin	These are stimulant laxatives but work very quickly in about half to one hour.	May leak out of anus and cause itching.

DRUGS FROM DOCTOR

Usually all those drugs available from the doctor can be bought from the chemist. If in doubt though, **ALWAYS** contact a doctor.

CONTRACEPTION

There are a variety of methods to prevent pregnancy. Below are listed the various types of contraceptive pills that are available. Other methods of contraception available are the cap, the diaphragm, the sponge and the sheath (condom). These are all barrier methods and the advice of a doctor should be consulted.

The Coil is a device placed in the womb which prevents the egg settling in the womb.

DRUGS FROM CHEMIST

Sheaths and contraceptive sponges are available over the counter.

DRUGS FROM DOCTOR

Drug	Information	Possible Side Effects
The Combined-Pill Fixed Doses —Eugynon 30 —Femodene —Minilyn —Minovlar —Ovran —Loestrin 20/30 —Microgynon 30 —Minulet	Contains two hormones and stops the production of eggs every month and prevents sperm entering the womb.	Breast tenderness and weight gain are usual.
Biphasic/Triphasic (variable dose) —BiNovum —Trinovum —Logynon —Trinordiol	These must be taken in the correct order as the amount of drug changes throughout the course to mimic the body.	As above.
Progestogen-only-Pill (POP) —Femulen —Micronor —Microval —Neogest	Contains only one hormone and prevents sperm from entering the womb and the womb from accepting the egg.	Irregular menstrual bleeding.
'Morning-After'-Pill (Schering PC4)	Taken after unprotected sexual intercourse. Contains a strong dose of two hormones. Prevents the egg from being accepted by the womb.	Sickness.

CONSULT YOUR DOCTOR OR PHARMACIST BEFORE TAKING MEDICATION

COUGHS (See also Colds)

A cough is the bodies way of getting rid of unwanted mucus. This mucus can come from the nose or the chest. Coughs can also be of the dry type where no mucus is involved. These dry 'tickly' coughs can be irritating and disturb sleep.

The medicines used to treat coughs can be broadly broken down into three groups. These are 1. Linctuses to soothe the throat. 2. Expectorants to make mucus more watery and therefore easier to cough up. 3. Cough suppressants to suppress a tickly and irritable cough.

The doses of all these three may be present in all or part in any cough medicine. However, although the expectorants and suppressants are only present in small amounts. If large doses are taken, then drowsiness may occur. Some medicines also contain antiseptics, antihistamines and painkillers in order to act as an all in one remedy. Ensure you don't double up doses by taking too many preparations.

Mucus can be loosened by use of simple steam or menthol inhalations. Sucking boiled sweets can be useful for dry tickly throats.

Most cough mixtures have very similar effects. There is little to choose between them in terms of effectiveness. The things to consider when buying a cough medicine are:

1. **What type of cough is it for?**
2. **Who is it for, child or adult?**
3. **Is the patient diabetic (i.e. must their sugar levels be controlled)**
4. **Will any drowsiness or sleepiness caused effect their work etc.?**
5. **Will any of the ingredients in the mixture upset the patients stomach, i.e. antiseptics.**
6. **Is the patient an asthmatic?**
7. **Price, the most expensive may not necessarily be the best.**

There are very many cough medicines, just a few are listed below. If in doubt it is best to consult your pharmacist. NOTE several large companies have their own brand name equivalents which are just as effective as the proprietary brands.

COUGHS *(continued)*

DRUGS FROM CHEMIST

Drug	Information	Possible Side Effects
Linctus/Honey and Lemon Mixtures. —Glycerin honey and lemon	Simply soothes the throat.	Diabetics should check with their GP that they can take these sugar-free preparations.
Cough Medicines —Cupal adult cough balm —Corona Bronchial Balsam —Pholcomed D Linctus	Usually contain one or more of the drugs that can be prescribed by the doctor. e.g. Decongestants, bronchodilators and cough suppressants	
—Adult Meltus; Expectorant Cough Linctus Dry Cough Elixir	For chesty coughs. For deep chesty coughs. Dry tickly coughs and catarrh.	
—Veno's Cough Mixture Expectorant Honey and Lemon	Dry cough. Chesty cough. Tickly cough (more a linctus).	
—Dimotane Expectorant —Congesteze Syrup —Bronalin Paediatric —Benylin Children sugar free	Coughs and congestion. As the name suggests sugar free.	
—Lotussin —Robitussin —Tixylix —Vapo syrup —Benylin	Cough Soother. Childrens coughs. Dry coughs. Varieties for chesty coughs, dry coughs.	
—Actifed Syrup Compound Linctus Expectorant —Sudafed Expectorant —Sudafed Linctus —Sudafed Elixir —Bronalin	Varieties for dry cough, expectorant.	

CONSULT YOUR DOCTOR OR PHARMACIST BEFORE TAKING MEDICATION

CRABS (see Parasites)

CRAMP (Painful spasm of body muscles)

Cramps are a very common condition and are more prevalent in some people than others. The elderly are especially prone. The cause is not exactly known but it seems possible that the depravation of certain types of salt to the muscles might be important. Heat, say a hot water bottle and rubbing the effected area to encourage blood flow can help. Alternatively an ice pack might help. Stretching or flexing of the muscle can help too.

DRUGS FROM CHEMIST

Drug	Information	Possible Side Effects
Crampex.	For night cramps.	Few.
Salt tablets.	Used in hot climates to replace lost salts.	Cause excessive thirst.

DRUGS FROM DOCTOR

Drug	Information	Possible Side Effects
Quinine bisulphate.	For night cramps taken before going to bed.	Few. Do not take more than prescribed.
Cyclandelate.	Prevents muscles from spasming by increasing circulation.	Nausea, flushing, in high doses.

CYSTITIS

This is a condition where passing urine becomes very frequent and painful. There is also a constant feeling of wanting to urinate. It is much more common in women than men. It is usually caused by an infection of the urethra, or less frequently the kidneys. It can help to avoid alcohol and wear loose underclothing. If it persists then consult a doctor.

DRUGS FROM CHEMIST (may also be prescribed by doctor)

Drug	Information	Possible Side Effects
Neutralising agents Potassium Citrate Citric Acid Effercitrate Sodium Bicarbonate Cystoleve	Neutralises the acid in patient's urine. Quite effective.	May cause sickness and nausea.

DRUGS FROM DOCTOR

Drug	Information	Possible Side Effects
Antibiotics: —Ampicillin; —Co-trimoxazole; —Fectrim; —Septrin; —Nitrofurantoin; —Nalidixic acid; —Mictral.	Most often used cure; works by killing the bacteria. If used in excess the bacteria may become resistant.	See General Side Effects. Certain drugs of this type should not be taken during pregnancy.

For more details on antibacterials and antibiotics, see these entries in the book.

CONSULT YOUR DOCTOR OR PHARMACIST BEFORE TAKING MEDICATION

DEAFNESS (See Ear Infections)

DEPRESSION

Most people probably feel depressed at some point in their lives. The word depression in fact may mean different things to different people. In general though it may be said to be a feeling of "downness", crying easily, lack of concentration and interest, low self-esteem. Feelings of hopelessness. It can last for just a few days or for very long periods.

In addition to the above symptoms, depression can also be an illness in itself which can be treated as a clinical disease. Most depression may well get better on it's own if left alone, but there are times treatment from the doctor is necessary. It's causes can vary. It can result from an emotional problem or may be due to a physical cause such as an upset in body chemistry.

DRUGS FROM CHEMIST

Anti-depressants are not sold over-the-counter. A doctor must always be consulted. Be careful with the herbal and homeopathic remedies. They have not been proven to work.

DRUGS FROM DOCTOR

Drug	Information	Possible Side Effects

Anti-depressants:
Tricyclic/Cyclic
  compounds
—Amitriptyline
  Domical
  Lentizol
  Tryptizol
—Butriptyline
  Evadyne
—Clomipramine
  Anafranil
—Desipramine
  Pertofran
—Dothiepin
  Prothiaden
—Doxepin
  Sinequan
—Imipramine
  Tofranil
	These take up to three or more weeks to have an effect. They work on the brain possibly by stimulating the production of certain chemicals.	Dry mouth; blurred vision; constipation; If you operate machinery or drive it might be important to take care for a few days. Other side effects are possible such as decreased sexual function.

DRUGS FROM DOCTOR *(continued)*

Drug	Information	Possible Side Effects
—Lofepramine Gamanil —Nortriptyline Allegron Aventyl —Protriptyline Concordin —Trimipramine Surmontil Other preparations are available.		
Monoaximine Oxidise Inhibitors (MHOI'S): —Phenelzine Nardil —Isocarboxazid Marplan —Tranylcypromine Parnate	These drugs are able to block the breakdown of certain chemicals in the body.	Dry mouth, constipation. Dizziness on standing. Difficulty in urination. Always card a MAOI card. Avoid cheese, meat extracts and all non prescription drugs unless with advice from GP or pharmacist.
Lithium Salts; **Lithium Carbonate;** **Lithium Citrate.**	Used for long term treatment Reduces episodes of depression.	Nausea; diarrhoea; increased thirst.

Other drugs are sometimes used. These include mild stimulants for the central nervous system and Amphetamines/cocaine.

IMPORTANT: When coming off those drugs, it is important to reduce the dose gradually. Always consult your doctor before stopping any prescribed treatment.

DIARRHOEA

This term is given to increased fluidity and frequency of bowel movements (stools). Can be due to a number of factors such as food poisoning, stress or as a side effect of other medication. If the condition lasts for several days or if a child is affected, ask a doctor for their advice. Ensure extra fluids are taken because diarrhoea causes dehydration. Eat bland food, but avoid milk and milk products. Women taking the Contraceptive pill should follow the advice of the manufacturer or their doctor for the condition might alter the effectiveness of the pill itself.

Treatment for the condition can be twofold. If the diarrhoea is caused by an infection then antibiotics might be taken. On the other hand if the cause is non infectious a drug to reduce the bowel movement might be useful. If the condition is accompanied by vomiting or in babies under two then medical help should be immediately sought. Always remember that it is important to drink lots of fluid to prevent dehydration.

DRUGS FROM CHEMIST (may also be prescribed by the doctor)

Drug	Information	Possible Side Effects
Anti-diarrhoeal drugs: Kaolin and Morphine Kaopectate Enterosan	These drugs do not prevent dehydration and should be used with care. They should not be used for more than three days consecutively. These drugs prevent bowel movements by acting on the gut contents.	Used to excess will cause constipation.
—Codeine Phosphate Kaodene	These drugs act on the wall of the gut to slow down its movement.	May cause constipation.
—Arret (loperamide/ Imodium —Diocalm	As above.	
Glucose-Salt Prescriptions: —Sodium Chloride; —Dioralyte; —Rehidrat. —Diocalm Junior	Extremely important in severe diarrhoea. Use in addition to the above. Replaces lost fluid and essential salts.	Can cause sickness or nausea. If this occurs try different type.

DRUGS FROM DOCTOR

Drug	Information	Possible Side Effects
Antibiotics: see ANTIBIOTICS	Antibiotics only really work for those forms of diarrhoea caused by bacteria. These must be taken for the time period specified.	See General Side Effects.
Anti-diarrhoeal drugs Lomotil Imodium (loperamide)	Will cause bowels movements to slow down and so reduce frequency of movements. Follow doctors instructions.	
Codeine phosphate —Diarrest	Acts on gut wall to slow down its movements.	Constipation.

DIZZINESS (Vertigo)

Dizziness is a sensation of loss of balance and movement of the patient or objects around them. The causes are many and a consistent attack of more than 24-hours should be investigated. Causes include drugs, inner ear problems, infections, blood pressure, low blood glucose and anxiety.

Travel Sickness is a form of this and some antihistamine travel sickness pills are available from the chemist.

DRUGS FROM CHEMIST (may also be prescribed by the doctor)

Some antihistamines, in the form of travel sickness pills can be bought from the chemist, but all general consistent dizzy spells should be investigated by a doctor.

DRUGS FROM DOCTOR

Drug	Information	Possible Side Effects
Tranquillisers —Diazepam. (valium)	Used for dizziness associated with tension.	Avoid alcohol. May cause drowsiness.
Antihistamines: —Prochlorperazine Stemitil Compazine Vertigon	These suppress or reduce the feeling of dizziness. Suppress the feeling of sickness, nausea and vertigo.	May cause blurred vision, dry mouth, constipation and should be avoided in pregnancy.

Ear Ache may be caused by an infection or wax build up. If the ear is infected see Ear Infections. However, it is often difficult to distinguish between the two, so after 2-3 days of ear ache **ALWAYS** seek medical attention. Flying can often cause short term ear pain.

DRUGS FROM CHEMIST (may also be prescribed by the Doctor)

Wax softening Drops: —Cerumol —Ear-ex —Wax-aid —Waxol; —Almond Oil	Softens the wax plug. The wax may then come out on its own. If a doctor has prescribed this then it may be used before syringing the ears.	May be messy. Be careful not to form a suction when applying as it may damage the ear drum. May irritate the ear.
Pain Killers: see PAIN	To relieve the pain of the ache. Do not use for more than a few days without consulting a doctor as to the cause.	See PAIN.

CONSULT YOUR DOCTOR OR PHARMACIST BEFORE TAKING MEDICATION

EAR INFECTIONS (See also Ear Ache)

This condition can be of two types. Those infections that occur inside the ear past the ear drum and those infections on the outside of the ear drum. Inner ear infections can cause dizziness, pain, sickness and discharge. External ear problems can also cause pain and discharge. Be aware of anything that might cause the problem, e.g. irritants such as shampoos, or a foreign body, especially in children.

DRUGS FROM CHEMIST (may also be prescribed by Doctor)

Drug	Information	Possible Side Effects
Pain Killers see PAIN.	Relieves pain. Should not be taken for several days without consulting a doctor to determine the cause.	see PAIN.

In all cases it is very dangerous to self-diagnose ear problems and a medical opinion should be sought if the pain does not go in 2 or 3 days.

DRUGS FROM DOCTOR

Drug	Information	Possible Side Effects
Antibiotic Drops See ANTIBIOTICS	These should be used as specified by a doctor.	
Antifungal drugs —Co-trimazole	To help combat fungal ear infections.	
—Decongestants Oral Psuedophedrine Actifed Sudafed	Can be given orally or as a nasal spray. These drugs help to relieve blockage.	Oral decongestants may cause insomnia. Take care in giving to children.
Nasal Otrivine Sinex Sinutab	As above.	May irritate the nose lining.
—Antihistamines	Help to combat allergies. May be mixed with a decongestant. Help reduce inflammation.	Most cause drowsiness.
—Steroids Prednisolone	Helps to reduce irritation and inflammation.	May mask secondary infections. Use over short periods.

28

ECZEMA

This is a condition describing red, itchy skin which can cause skin to thicken after years of intense scratching. Can be caused by allergic reactions to certain materials. Also can occur for no apparent external cause.

Types of Eczema:
1. Atopic — Often develops in childhood and may be associated with asthma and hayfever.
2. Discoid — Occurs in mid-adulthood and is found in circular patches on the limbs.
3. Varicose — Found on the legs.
4. Seborrheic — Type of endogenous eczema that causes flaking on the chest, scalp, face, eyebrows and eyelids.
5. Contact — Sensitivity to contact with certain substances such as detergents. Allergy based.

DRUGS FROM CHEMIST

Drug	Information	Possible Side Effects

—Moisturisers:
—Aqueous Cream
  Boots E45 Cream
  plus other
  preparations
—Bath Oils
	Very important in helping to keep the skin moist.	Irritation or allergic reactions.

—Shampoos (Anti-dandruff)	Helps stop itching on the scalp (Seborrheic Eczema).	

DRUGS FROM DOCTOR

Drug	Information	Possible Side Effects
Steroid ointments: —Dermovate; —Betnovate; —Eumovate; —Hydrocortisone.	Reduce inflammation and heal skin. Range of strengths exist.	Cause thinning of skin and so skin is easily bruised. Apply sparingly.
Antihistamines. See ANTIHISTAMINES	Reduce the itching and can help people to sleep.	Causes drowsiness.

CONSULT YOUR DOCTOR OR PHARMACIST BEFORE TAKING MEDICATION

EYE PROBLEMS

CONJUNCTIVITIS

There is also a viral form of conjunctivitis, which the antibiotics will have no effect on. However this clears up within two to three weeks on it's own.

DRUGS FROM CHEMIST

None available. Any over-the-counter treatments should only be used after taking doctor's advice.

DRUGS FROM DOCTOR

Drug	Information	Possible Side Effects
Antibiotics —Chloramphenicol —Gentamicin —Neomycin. SEE ANTIBIOTICS	Antibiotics used to kill bacteria in either eye drops or ointment form.	Can blur vision for short while so don't drive until it has cleared. Allergic reactions may occur.

BLEPHRITIS

There are two forms of Belphritis. The bacterial form causes ulceration of the eye lid and the squamous form, which causes flaky skin on the eyelashes. It is often a long term condition.

DRUGS FROM CHEMIST

None available. Any over-the-counter treatments should only be used after taking doctor's advice. Medicated shampoo's may help the squamous form of Blephritis.

DRUGS FROM DOCTOR

Drug	Information	Possible Side Effects
Antibiotics	Antibiotics used to kill bacteria.	Can blur vision for short while.

FLU (Influenza)

This is a viral infection experienced by most people at some time or another. It is very infectious and is particularly common in the colder months of the year. The symptoms hardly need describing, suffice to say they are very similar to the common cold. There is a definite feeling of 'grottiness' and being unwell. However in the old, very young and the ill the condition can become very serious, turning into more serious diseases such as pneumonia.

DRUGS FROM CHEMIST

Fuller details can be found in the entry on the Colds, but briefly the following types of drugs and treatments can be bought at a pharmacy.

Drug	Information	Possible Side Effects
Pain Killers —Paracetamol —Aspirin	Mainly reduce pain and lower body temperature. They should be repeated fairly regularly. Aspirin is slightly more effective.	Do not give Aspirin to children under 12.
Decongestants —Pseudoephedrine —Actifed —Sudafed	Dry up secretions and reduce swelling in the nasal passage.	

DRUGS FROM DOCTOR

Drug	Information	Possible Side Effects
Antibiotics See ANTIBIOTICS	Prevents secondary infection. These should only be used sparingly to prevent resistance building up.	

FUNGAL INFECTIONS

Fungal infections include Thrush (also known as Candida), Athletes Foot and Ringworm. Babies Nappy Rash may also be a form of Thrush. Fungal infections are caused by mould-like organisms which live on the skin. Fungi thrive best in warm moist conditions and so are found most commonly under the arms, between the legs, between the toes and in the mouth. Different fungi can live in different places on the body causing different conditions. Fungal infections are not usually serious but can last a long time.

Fungal infections can be caught from animals, and a few such as athletes foot, can be caught from humans. The onset of infections such as Thrush (candida) can appear to be due to no particular cause, just perhaps being a little run down. Other times the cause can be specifically identified.

DRUGS FROM CHEMIST

Always see a doctor in the event of these complaints occurring. Although regular washing can help. See also Athletes Foot.

Drug	Information	Possible Side Effects
Daktarin Oral Gel	Useful for oral thrush. Follow instructions exactly.	None
Canesten Cream	An antifungal cream. Ensure infection is fungal before beginning treatment.	

DRUGS FROM DOCTOR

Drug	Information	Possible Side Effects
Imidazole: —Econazole: —Miconazole: —Clotrimazole: —Nystatin plus others	Used as a cream. Used for many fungal infections.	May all cause allergies. They may allow secondary infections to develop.
—Griseofulvin: —Ketoconazole.	Used for nail infections.	Ketoconazole may cause liver damage.
Whitfields ointment.	Becoming out of date.	

These drugs may be delivered as lotions, creams, sprays or ointments or dusting powders.

GASTROENTERITIS

This is a condition which can cause several nasty symptoms. These include diarrhoea (frequent passing of loose or liquid faeces), a painful tummy, vomiting and a general feeling of feeling poorly. It is usually caused by infective bacteria, viruses or food poisons. These are very often caught by eating 'bad' or infected food which may be the cause of the food poisoning. There are two main types of gastroenteritis, one starts at about 2-4 hours and lasts for 12-24 hours. The other type occurs about 8-12 hours after and lasts for 24-48 hours. See also Diarrhoea

DRUGS FROM CHEMIST

Drug	Information	Possible Side Effects
Glucose Salt Solution	Prevents dehydration. Seek doctor's advice for children.	Slight nausea.
Loperamide (Imodium, Arret) Kaolin and Morphine.	Relieve painful spasms, reduce frequency of diarrhoea.	Constipation if taken for too long.

DRUGS FROM DOCTOR

Drug	Information	Possible Side Effects
Glucose Salt Solution.	Prevents dehydration.	Slight nausea.
Anti-diarrhoearal drugs; —Codeine phosphate —Loperamide (Arret/Imodium) —Kaolin and Morphine.	Relieve painful spasms, reduce frequency of diarrhoea.	Constipation if taken for too long.
Antibiotics See ANTIBIOTICS	Kill bacteria.	

CONSULT YOUR DOCTOR OR PHARMACIST BEFORE TAKING MEDICATION

HAY FEVER

Hay fever is an allergic reaction of the body to some form of 'allergen'. These allergens are most commonly various types of pollen from trees and plants. It is these pollens that can trigger the release of a chemical called histamine which then causes the symptoms. The symptoms are very distressing to the sufferer and may include a runny nose, sneezing and watering of the eyes.

DRUGS FROM CHEMIST

Drug	Information	Possible Side Effects
Decongestants (eye and nose) —Oxymetazoline —Ephedrine Nasal drops —Xylometazoline Otrivine. Sinex Nasal Spray	Available as eye drops or nasal spray. Give temporary relief.	Continued use will irritate nose and enhance symptoms of hay fever.
Antihistamine —Astemizole —Chlorpheniramine —Clemastine; —Terfenadine (Triludan).	These are antihistamines and are used both in short and long term to stop histamine production. See Antihistamines.	Drowsiness. DO NOT DRINK OR DRIVE if affected. Dry mouth. See Antihistamines.

DRUGS FROM DOCTOR

Drug	Information	Possible Side Effects
Antihistamines See above		
Steroids: —Prednisolone.	Used for short periods only to block allergic reactions. Very effective.	Safe if used for a **short** time only.
Nasal sprays: —Steroid sprays: Beclomethasone; Budesonide.	Reduce symptoms during an attack and are taken for long periods to stop allergic reactions.	No significant effects for sprays.
Sodium Cromoglycate. —Rynacrom	Reduce symptoms during an attack and are taken for long periods to stop allergic reactions.	No significant effects for sprays.
Decongestants See above		

HIATUS HERNIA (OESOPHAGITIS)

We all have a tube (the oesophagus) which reaches from the mouth to the stomach. It is down this that our food travels. There is a small valve at the point where the oesophagus meets the top of the stomach. This is called the cardiac sphincter. Sometimes, when things go wrong, the walls of the stomach can actually push up through the hole in a membrane called the diaphram, which allows the tube through to meet the stomach. The subsequent distortion of the stomach wall can cause problems with the function of the small valve. This is then called a hiatus hernia.

The symptoms are usually heartburn and an unpleasant taste in the mouth. It may also cause a feeling of burning pain in the chest.

A related condition is Oesophagitis where the gullet becomes inflamed.

DRUGS FROM CHEMIST

Drug	Information	Possible Side Effects
Antacids —Actal Tabs —Magnesium Trisil. —Gaviscon —Aludrox —Rennie Gold —Rennie Rapeze —Settlers —Ovals —Sovol —Bisodol —Asilone —Maalox —Milk of Magnesia	These can be used without prescription but continual use should be avoided and you should seek help from a doctor. These drugs neutralise the acid in the stomach.	Avoid Aluminium (causes constipation). Magnesium (causes diarrhoea). Sodium drugs (cause hypertension or where reduced sodium diet has been advised.

Cont . . .

CONSULT YOUR DOCTOR OR PHARMACIST BEFORE TAKING MEDICATION

DRUGS FROM DOCTOR

Drug	Information	Possible Side Effects
Antacids See Above	These work by neutralizing the acid in the stomach which causes the pain.	Any aluminium drugs may cause constipation.

H2 Antagonists:
—Tagamet
  Cimetidine.
—Ranitidine
  Zantac
	They reduce the acid output of the stomach.	Cimetidine may interfere with other drugs.

Anti-emetics: —Prochlorperazine —Metoclopramide	These relieve the feeling of sickness.	Also avoid aluminium/magnesium sodium drugs as above.

INDIGESTION

Pain in the upper chest under the ribs. Can be combined with heartburn which is a burning sensation in the centre of the chest. Caused by inflammation of the stomach due to particular foods, alcohol, drugs and/or stress.

DRUGS FROM CHEMIST

There are a variety of proprietary antacids available all of which will act similar to those above from the doctor. Note: if you have continuous need for antacids and food also seems to help the pain, then see your doctor, as you may have an ulcer.

Drug	Information	Possible Side Effects
Antacids —Actal Tabs —Magnesium Trisil. —Gaviscon —Aludrox	These work by neutralizing the acid in the stomach which causes the pain. These can be used without prescription but continual use should be avoided and you should seek help from a doctor.	Any aluminium drugs may cause constipation. Magnesium antacids may cause diarrhoea
—Rennie Gold —Rennie Rapeze —Settlers —Ovals —Sovol —Bisodol —Asilone —Maalox —Milk of Magnesia	Can be purchased as liquids or chewable tablets	Avoid sodium containing drugs.

DRUGS FROM DOCTOR

Drug	Information	Possible Side Effects
Antacids: See above	Available as liquid or chewable tablets; coat stomach and neutralise acid.	Aluminium antacids cause constipation. Magnesium antacids cause diarrhoea.

Anti-emetics:
—Metoclopramide;
  Maxolon
  Gastrobid
  Domperidone.
	Lessen the pain and nausea.	

CONSULT YOUR DOCTOR OR PHARMACIST BEFORE TAKING MEDICATION

Prevention is probably better than cure when it's come to such problems. The main way of preventing bites and stings is to use some form of insect repellant. These are now available as lotions, creams, sprays and wipes.

If you are bitten, calamine lotion is a very effective soothing agent. Certain people are allergic to bee and wasp stings and should consult a doctor if this is known to be the case. Immunisation is sometimes required. This is especially true when travelling abroad. If you are allergic to bee stings it is important to carry an antihistamine tablet with you ready in case you should be stung. There might not be time to get to a doctor if this does happen. It usually takes about half an hour for the allergic reaction to take effect.

DRUGS FROM CHEMIST

Drug	Information	Possible Side Effects
Insect Repellents —Oil of Lavender —Shoo —Combat —Jungle —Dusk	Very Effective	None.
Dimethyl phthalate —Sketofax		
Dibutyl phthalate	Used to impregnate clothing lasts for two weeks even with washing. May produce hypersensitivity.	
Insect Bite Creams —Swarm —RBC cream —Afterbite	There are many available. Ask your pharmacist for the best one for you. These may contain antihistamines.	These may cause further skin irritation.
Antihistamines	Although also available from the doctor, there are many also obtainable from the pharmacist. See Antihistamines.	Can cause drowsiness.

INSECT BITES AND STINGS *(continued)*

DRUGS FROM DOCTOR

Drug	Information	Possible Side Effects
Antihistamines —Promethazine	May be given by injection for immediate relief.	
Steroid/Adrenalin —Hydrocortisone and others	Maybe given by injection to alleviate severe allergic reactions.	None in the short term.

ITCHING

The desire to persistently scratch can be caused by a number of factors. Skin disorders such as eczema and psoriasis as well as Chickenpox can be a major irritation. Allergic reactions and insect bites can also be 'itchy'. An itch in a particular area can indicate another problem, e.g. if around the anus it may indicate say haemorrhoids, or alternatively vaginal irritation may be due to a localized infection. Each cause may result in a different remedy depending on the reason for the irritation.

DRUGS FROM CHEMIST

Drug	Information	Possible Side Effects
Soothing and cooling preparations —Aqueous Cream —Calamine lotion —Cold cream	Useful for mild itching such as sunburn and insect bites. Aqueous cream will soothe dry skin.	None.
Local Anaesthetics —Lignocaine —Benzocaine Lanocane	Useful for small areas of itching caused by sunburn, insect bites, allergic reactions.	May cause allergic reaction.
Haemorrhoid Treatment See Piles	For anal itching.	
Local Antihistamines —RBC (Antazoline) —Anthisan (Mepyramine) —Swarm A	These are useful for small areas such as insect bites and nettle rash.	May cause allergic reactions.
Oral Antihistamines —Piriton	Useful for insect bites and allergic reactions.	May cause drowsiness.

DRUGS FROM DOCTOR

Drug	Information	Possible Side Effects
Local Corticorsteroids —Hydrocortisone	Useful for inflammatory skin complaints especially eczema. Very effectve in other conditions. Should not be used on a long term basis.	Do not use for long periods.

LICE (See Parasites)

MEASLES (See Childrens Ailments)

MENOPAUSAL PROBLEMS

These occur at the time in a womens life when she ceases to be able to bear children. This age can vary, but it is usually between 45 to 55. Though it can be outside this age group. The symptoms may include hot sweats, aching limbs, dry/sore vagina, thin bones etc.

DRUGS FROM CHEMIST

Drug	Information	Possible Side Effects
Calcium Tablets	These help stop bones thinning. They are of limited use.	None.

DRUGS FROM DOCTOR

Drug	Information	Possible Side Effects
Hormone replacement Therapy (HRT) Oestrogen.	These help balance the woman's hormones as the natural levels in her body change. These can be taken as tablets or as a vaginal cream. Also as an implant for women who have not had hysterectomy. Progesterone is included for some time every month to reduce the chance of cancer.	There is a slight possibility of illness if not taken properly. So always discuss any past illnesses and conditions with the doctor before taking any HRT treatment.

MENSTRUAL PROBLEMS (Period Pains)

Period problems can be one or a mixture of types. This can include heavy periods, infrequent periods, painful periods and often the very distressing pre-menstrual-tension. (PMT). This can include fluid retention, bloating, tension and irritability.

DRUGS FROM CHEMIST

Drug	Information	Possible Side Effects
Mild Painkiller See Pain	Helps with the pain and muscle spasms.	Consult doctor before taking these medicines.
Vitamin B6 —Benadon	May help reduce period symptoms. Usual dose is 50mg or 100mg per day during period.	

DRUGS FROM DOCTOR

Drug	Information	Possible Side Effects
Hormones such as Oestrogen and Progesterone	This helps to re-balance the hormone levels in the body and reduce the symptoms.	These may cause weight gain, fluid retention and nausea and/or headache. Acne.
Prostaglandin Inhibitors: —Mefenamic Acid (Ponstan)	Reduces heavy periods.	Dizziness and nausea.
Antispasmodic Drugs —Buscopan	These reduce painful periods by relaxing the muscles.	Dry mouth and palpitations.
Diuretics There are a variety of types	Help reduce water retention.	Just possibly gout.
Antifibrinolytic Drugs: —Amcar and others	Reduce bleeding.	Nausea.
Analgesics/ Painkillers	Reduces the pain of periods.	See Pain killers.

MOUTH ULCERS

These are painful ulcers found in the mouth and on the tongue. Although only minor in severity, they can be very painful indeed and make eating very unpleasant. There are various types of mouth ulcers and sometimes they are caused by more serious conditions. So if they persist for more than a week or so, you should consult your doctor.

DRUGS FROM CHEMIST

Drug	Information	Possible Side Effects
Pastilles —Rinstead —ulc-aid	Soothes mouth and ulcer.	None.
Antiseptic Mouthwashes/ treatments —Corsodyl —Hibitane —Medigel —Anbesol —Ulcaid —J Pickles mouth treatment	As above.	

DRUGS FROM DOCTOR

Drug	Information	Possible Side Effects
Antibiotics Nystatin —Nystan —Fungelin **See Antibiotics and Antifungals**	Helps clear up any bacterial or fungal infections. Used for Thrush. Usually given as lozenges, gels or creams.	May cause nausea.
Steroids	Used for more severe mouth ulcers.	None in the short term.
Iron Tablets	For mouth ulcers caused by anaemia.	

CONSULT YOUR DOCTOR OR PHARMACIST BEFORE TAKING MEDICATION

NAPPY RASH

Nappy rash can usually be seen as a red rash around the nappy area and this can extend from the waist to the knee. Nappy rash can be caused by a fungal infection and is then known as Thrush. The appearance of red spots at the edge of the rash is the usual tell tale sign of it's presence. Thrush is caused by the yeast Candida albicans.

Other forms of Nappy rash can be caused by an irritant dermatitis (due to urine or faecies being held in the warm, damp nappy). Alternatively it can be due to an allergic reaction caused by a detergent or soap powder. Finally fever, teething or antibiotic treatment could all be a cause.

If nappy rash occurs it is best to check that you have not recently changed soap powders or detergents and so that an allergic reaction is not a possibility. Also changing from a different make of disposable nappy may occasionally be a cause.

Preventative Measures:
1.   Wash and Rinse Nappies Well, use non-allergic detergent.
2.   Leave nappy off the baby for an hour or so at a time.

DRUGS FROM DOCTOR

Drug	Information	Possible Side Effects
Preventative:	Acts as a barrier to irritant. Also	Can be messy
Vaseline	soothes skin.	
Sudocrem	As above.	
Zinc and Castor Oil	As above.	
Dimethicone	These three preparations contain	Do not use on open
Siopel	silicone which acts as a barrier to	sores or broken skin.
Vasogen.	prevent irritation.	
Antiseptics:	Help to clean an area once nappy	Take care as may cause
Cetrimide	rash has occurred. Drapolene has	an allergic or sensitive
Drapolene	some anti-fungal properties.	skin reaction.

DRUGS FROM DOCTOR

An Antibiotic may be used to tackle a fungal infection, see section on antibiotics. Possibly a corticosteroid such as hydrocortisone cream might be used in severe cases. Always consult the doctor if the problem does not clear up.

NERVOUS TENSION (See Anxiety)

PAINKILLERS (Analgesic)

Pain killers can vary in their strength and in their mode of action. The site of action of a pain killer is also an important point to bear in mind when selecting one to relieve an area of pain. For instance an Non-steroidal anti-inflammatory (NSAID), such as Aspirin, is able to reduce the swelling and inflammation around a site of pain. Thus a weaker NSAID might well be more effective than a stronger dose of say paracetamol in certain circumstances.

Below is a rough guide to the relative strengths of pain killers available from the pharmacist and doctor. It has to be said though that the selection of such a drug will depend as much on the type of pain and its location as the strength of the pain killer itself. For details on each drug see the entry in the main text.

ORDER OF STRENGTH IN PAIN KILLERS

(weakest)

1. *Chemist (across the counter)* **painkillers**

Aspirin/Paracetamol/Ibuprofen — All about the same strength although the extra or stronger varieties may be more effective). The most powerful over the counter painkillers are:

Solpadeine

Propain

Panadeine

2. *Painkillers only available on* **prescription** *from the Doctor*

Antagonists
e.g. Pentazocine — Quite strong, certainly more so than over the counter pain killers. However these are less effective than morphine, but less addictive.

Morphine Derivatives
e.g. Dihydrocodeine — More effective than the antagonists, but still not the strongest.

Morphine/Narcotics
e.g. Diamorphine (Heroin) — Strongest painkillers available, but can cause severe side effects.

(Strongest)

Cont . . .

There are three major types of painkillers (analgesic) available from your chemist.

Note: Although Codeine also exists as an over the counter painkiller, the doses are so small as to be of limited value in relieving pain. It can only be obtained in effective doses by prescription from the doctor. It can be included in other painkillers.

DRUGS FROM CHEMIST

Drug	Information	Possible Side Effects
Paracetamol: —Anadin paracetamol —Disprol —Hedex —Panadol —Paraclear —Paracets	Relieves pain and reduces temperature. Does not upset the stomach and is suitable for people with ulcers. However it has no anti-inflammatory action and you must not exceed the stated daily dose.	Overdose can be dangerous—seek medical help. Long term use together with regular alcohol intake may cause liver damage.
Paracetamol combinations: —Co-codamol —Panadeine —Propain —Triogesic	These preparations contain codeine, another painkiller to make a stronger pain relieve.	If taken regularly codeine can cause constipation.
—Disprin Extra* —Anadin Extra* —Panadol Extra* —Veganin*	*These also contain aspirin.	See side effects of both aspirin and paracetamol.
Aspirin: —Anadin —Anadin extra —Askit —Aspro —Aspro clear —Aspro clear extra —Codis —Disprin —Disprin Extra —Equagesic —Migraclear Migraleve Veganin	Has both painkilling effect and anti-inflammatory actions. Which means it will help reduce the swelling which might be responsible for the pain in the first place. An example of this would be an abscess on a tooth root which can cause intense pain. Not to be taken by children under 12.	Can cause stomach irritation. Do not take if you suffer from stomach trouble or ulcers. It may cause internal bleeding. Asthmatics should avoid aspirin. Excessive doses of aspirin may cause ringing in the ears and nausea. It is possible to develop an allergic reaction to aspirin.

46

DRUGS FROM CHEMIST *(continued)*

Drug	Information	Possible Side Effects
Ibuprofen Anadin/Ibuprofen —Cuprofen —Ibuleve (gel) —Nurofen —Proflex —Inoven —Librofem	Similar to aspirin it has the ability to reduce swelling and inflammation as well as give pain relief.	Has similar side effects to Aspirin, should not be given to people with ulcers.

DRUGS FROM DOCTOR

There are two main classes of drug that the doctor can prescribe. These are:

CLASS 1   Morphine or Narcotic derivatives.—The most potent painkillers available to prescribe. The side effects however can be quite severe.

Morphine Derivatives.—Less effective but cause less severe side effects.

CLASS 2   Antagonist—Least strong, but still quite potent compared to drugs from the chemist. Side effects can be distressing for some people even though they are not as bad as the other prescription pain killers.

The main distinction in these powerful analgesic is between the drugs that are controlled drugs (CD) because of their power such as Heroin and Morphine and those that might well be of the same class but are slightly less potent (such as Co-proxamol).

Drug	Information	Possible Side Effects
CLASS 1		
Morphine/Narcotics —MST Continus —Nepenthe —Cyclimorph	Only lasts for a short period of time, therefore need frequent dosing except when using MST tablets.	Nausea and vomiting are common. May cause addiction.

Cyclimorph contains an anti-emetic which helps reduce the nausea side effect.

Cont...

CLASS 1 *(continued)*

Drug	Information	Possible Side Effects
Related drugs —Opium —Pethidine —Diamorphine (Heroin) —Methadone	These drugs are very strong and are only used with caution. Sometimes used as a Heroin substitute for the treatment of addiction.	Must be given with extreme caution to patients with breathing problems as it may depress breathing centres in brain.

All of the above drugs are CD or controlled drugs. These drugs are mostly VERY addictive and have very strict controls on their prescription.

Dextropropoxyphene —Co-Proxamol —Distalgesic	Useful painkillers for mild to moderate pain. Also contain paracetamol.	
Morphine Derivatives —Codeine Phosphate —Dihydrocodeine DF 118 —Paracodol —Co-dydramol —Co-codamol	Useful for moderate pain relief. Should not be used on a long term basis as may cause constipation. Dihydrocodeine/paracetamol mixture. A mixture of codeine and paracetamol.	May cause constipation, dizziness, vomiting, and drowsiness. Musn't be given to patients with respiratory illness. Not so addictive.

CLASS 2

Antagonists —Pentazocine Fortral Fortagesic		May cause dizziness and constipation. Very similar to Codeine.
—Buprenorphine Temgesic	Much less addictive than other narcotics. Useful for moderate to severe pain.	Similar to morphine, but less pronounced side effects.

These drugs are both CD's

Other drugs
—NSAIDS
  Ibuprofen
  Diclofenac
  Fenbufen´
    (Lederfen)
  Indomethacin
  Ketoprofen
    (Alrheumat)
  Mefenamic acids
    (Ponstan)
  Naproxen
    (Naprosyn)
  Piroxicam
    (Feldene)
  Tiaprofenic acid
    (Surgam)

Often used in rheumatic disease or other muscular disorders.

Asthmatics should not take NSAIDS except on doctors advice. Avoid with peptic ulcers.

NOTE: Many drugs contain mixtures of other active ingredients. For instance aspirin is found in many cold remedies. Therefore make sure if you take a pain killer such as aspirin for pain relief that you do not inadvertently take a double dose with a secondary medicine taken for a different reason.

CONSULT YOUR DOCTOR OR PHARMACIST BEFORE TAKING MEDICATION

PARASITES (Scabies, Nits, Crabs, Body Lice)

These are small organisms which live on human hair or skin. Scabies live under the skin, commonly found on hands, or genitals. Body lice are often found in clothes and all over the body. Lice (Nits) live on the hair. Crabs live on pubic hair. They may all cause itching.

DRUGS FROM CHEMIST

Most of the drugs available from the doctor are available from the chemist.

Drug	Information	Possible Side Effects
SCABIES		There may be some skin irritation.
Benzyl Benzoate —Ascabiol	The lotion is applied all over the body, except for the head and neck. Always follow the makers instructions closely.	
Monosulfiram —Tetmosol		
Lindane —Esoderm. —Lorexane —Derbac Soap —Quellada —Scabex	Always consult a doctor if the infestation continues. These preparations will NOT work unless they are used properly.	
NITS AND LICE **Malathion** —Prioderm —Suleo-M —Derbac	Mostly used as lotions. Ensure the instructions are followed closely. Comb hair with a fine tooth comb to remove lice and eggs.	Some preparations contain inflammable substances and should be used with care near naked flames.
Carbaryl —Carylderm —Clinicide		
CRABS —Malathion		
Carbanyl Lindane —Quellada		

DRUGS FROM DOCTOR

Drug	Information	Possible Side Effects
—Eurax Cream	Helps prevent itching whilst treatment works. Can also be bought from chemist.	Avoid broken skin.

PILES (Haemorrhoids)

This condition occurs when veins just inside the anus become swollen and irritated. This can be caused by pregnancy, or by sitting down for very long periods. The condition is made worse by constipation and straining. They can occasionally bleed slightly with extreme pain and must be seen by a doctor in these cases.

DRUGS FROM CHEMIST

Drug	Information	Possible Side Effects
Soothing agents: —Anusol —Germoloids —Preparation H	These soothe the affected area and relieve symptoms. This allows the haemorrhoid to return to normal with time.	May cause irritation.
—Hemocane	Contains a local anaesthetic to aid pain relief. Soothing agents also included.	May cause irritation.
Laxatives: see CONSTIPATION	These can ensure that stools are soft and so avoid straining which can make haemorrhoids worse.	Should not be used on a long term basis.

DRUGS FROM DOCTOR

Drug	Information	Possible Side Effects
Steroid creams Anugesic HC Anusol HC	These creams contain an agent which relieves inflammation around the anus. These often contain soothing agents also.	Do not use for prolonged periods as may cause reddening of the skin.
Local Anaesthetic —Lignocaine	These cause local numbness to relieve the pain.	

SCARLET FEVER (See Childrens Ailments)

CONSULT YOUR DOCTOR OR PHARMACIST BEFORE TAKING MEDICATION

SHINGLES (Herpes Zoster)

An infection caused by the same virus as chicken pox. It causes a painful, itchy rash on the skin with the appearance of small blisters. Nausea, lethargy and loss of appetite often occur. It may last for several months.

DRUGS FROM CHEMIST

Drug	Information	Possible Side Effects
Painkillers. —Paracetamol —Aspirin	Relieve pain. This is especially true in older patients where the pain may be so intense and over such a long period that simple painkillers may not be enough. Depression may set in if the condition is not managed properly.	Do not use unless checked with doctor.
Calamine Lotion.	Soothes and cools skin.	None.

DRUGS FROM DOCTOR

Drug	Information	Possible Side Effects
Antiviral agents: Idoxuridine; Acyclovir.	Must be applied locally as cream/ointment to reduce pain. Have limited use and effectiveness.	Can cause stinging of skin. Also redness and drying of skin with over-use.
Simple Analgesics: Paracetamol; Aspirin; Ibuprofen; Naproxen sodium. Co-Proxamol DF118 Detropropoxyphene	Reduces pain. Stronger pain killers only available on prescription, such as DF118's and Co-proxamol may be necessary.	See Side Effects of Pain.
Lotions: Calamine Lotion.	Cools and soothes skin.	None.

SICKNESS and TRAVEL SICKNESS

Sickness and nausea is the desire to lose food from the stomach through the mouth. This feeling is controlled from an area in the brain. It can also be just an awful feeling in the stomach and/or an all over feeling of general bad health and being unwell.

Travel sickness is a variation on this, which is brought about when travelling in some form of vehicle. Often a car, coach, train or plane. The symptoms here in addition to feeling sick can include dizziness, feeling flushed and sweating.

Continual vomiting can cause dehydration and this must be reversed by taking lots of fluids in such a situation. The causes for feelings of sickness can be many, but if the feeling or actual vomiting continues for more than a few days then a doctors help must be sought.

DRUGS FROM CHEMIST (may also be prescribed by the doctor)

Drug	Information	Possible Side Effects
Rehydration Fluids: —Dextrolyte; —Rehydrat.	Keeps water levels in the body at sufficient level.	
Glucose-Salt Solution	Helps to rehydrate the body.	
Travel Sickness Pills —Quells —Joy-Rides —Dramamine —Sturgeon —Marzine	These help to reduce the feeling of sickness in the centre of the brain that controls such feelings. They are often antihistamines (See Antihistamines) Take before leaving on the journey (check with the packet).	Drowsiness. Dry mouth.

DRUGS FROM DOCTOR

Drug	Information	Possible Side Effects
Antiemetic Drugs: —Stemetil —Stugeron —Evoxin —Vertigon	These are used ony for persistent vomiting rather than odd feelings of sickness. They work by blocking the part of the brain which gives the sensation of sickness. Some such as Cinnarzine are used for Travel Sickness.	These may cause drowsiness (made worse by alcohol). Also there may be headaches and irritability. Should not be used by people who have Glaucoma.

CONSULT YOUR DOCTOR OR PHARMACIST BEFORE TAKING MEDICATION

STINGS (See Insect Bites and Stings)

STRESS (See Anxiety)

SUNBURN

Sunburn is caused by too much exposure to sunlight. It can cause redness and soreness and great discomfort. Pain, heat and blistering of affected area may also occur.

DRUGS FROM CHEMIST

Drug	Information	Possible Side Effects
Sunscreens	Protect against sunburn by filtering out the harmful rays. The sun protection factor determines the degree of protection. (SPF).	None.
Calamine Lotion	Soothes itching and cools skin.	None.
Steroidal Creams	Soothes inflammation.	See Hydrocortisone below.
Painkillers	Aspirin and Paracetamol may work to reduce the pain. See Painkillers.	Do not give Aspirin to children under 12 years of age.

DRUGS FROM DOCTOR

Drug	Information	Possible Side Effects
Hydrocortisone Cream —Dioderm plus others.	For severe sunburn. This is a steroid cream.	Used only for a short time therefore no side effects.
Antihistamine Creams —Chlorphenizamine —Promethazine	Soothe itching and irritation.	Possible skin irritation.

SPRAINS

This definition would include strains and sprains of muscles, tendons, ligaments and joints. These injuries are usually felt as either severe or nagging pains or aches. Always keep the area warm and well supported. Perhaps try strapping the strain up with a tubular elasticated bandage.

DRUGS FROM CHEMIST

Drug	Information	Possible Side Effects
Mild Analgesics; NSAID's —Aspirin —Paracetamol —Ibuprofen	These can be bought from the chemist. The NSAIDS (Aspirin and ibuprofen) reduce the swelling and inflammation. See PAINKILLERS.	Do not give aspirin to children under 12 years of age.
Rubifactants —Algepan —Deep Heat —Wintergreen ointment	These are agents used to rub in or sprayed onto a troubled area. They cause a feeling of warmth in the skin which detracts from the pain felt. It is not proven that they have any lasting effect on deep pain.	See below.

DRUGS FROM DOCTOR

Drug	Information	Possible Side Effects
Analgesics: e.g. Aspirin; Paracetamol; etc. (See Pain)	Reduce the pain of the injury.	Codeine can cause nausea and constipation. Aspirin can cause Allergy.
NSAID's: e.g. Ibuprofen	These reduce swelling and tenderness and increase the speed of healing.	Similar to Aspirin.
Steroids.	Given as injections they reduce localised inflammation.	Can lead to tissue damage.
Rubifactants. See above.	These cause a warm feeling which tends to hide the pain.	May give allergic reactions if used on broken skin.

CONSULT YOUR DOCTOR OR PHARMACIST BEFORE TAKING MEDICATION

THRUSH (See Fungal Infections)

TOOTHACHE

Painkillers may be used on a very short term basis (See Painkillers). Tinctures are available from the chemist too. But the best treatment is from the Dentist. A 24-hour service is usually available from Teaching Hospitals. Also consult your Yellow pages for 24 hour dentists.

Stronger Painkillers, if prescribed, can be more effective than the mild analgesics.

Abscesses

If an abscess has developed on the root of the tooth (i.e. an infection) then it is the pressure of the pus building up around the root and pressing on the nerve which is causing much of the pain. This is especially likely if the tooth is broken or decayed. A dentist will not remove a tooth when this is the case. They will prescribe a common antibiotic (See Antibiotics) and give painkillers until the infection has cleared up.

NSAID pain killers are best here since they reduce the inflammation which is helping to cause the pain. These include Aspirin, Ibuprofen and all of their variants. (Again see Painkillers for more details).

The best treatment to reduce the pain if an abscess is diagnosed is to remain calm, (stress causes your blood pressure to rise and make things worse), keep it warm with a hot water bottle and take regular doses of your painkiller. Always try to take the painkillers before the pain takes a hold.

TONSILLITIS

This is an infection of the tonsils due to viral or bacterial infection. Symptoms usually include a sore throat and a general feeling of being unwell. Also fever and extreme difficulty in swallowing.

DRUGS FROM CHEMIST

The standard Cold Remedies may help reduce the symptoms. Painkillers may help (especially if gargled) and rest is essential. See entries on Colds and sore throats.

DRUGS FROM DOCTOR

Drug	Information	Possible Side Effects
Antibiotics: —Ampicillin; —Erythromycin etc.	If the cause is bacterial the antibiotics will destroy the bacteria, but in viral infections the antibiotics only prevent secondary infection.	Usual antibiotic side effects may occur.

TRAVEL SICKNESS (See Sickness)

ULCERS (Gastro-Intestinal)

Ulcers are breaks in the lining of the gastro-intestinal tract (G.I. Tract) which do not heal. This may lead to inflammation and possibly bleeding. G.I. tract ulcers can be of two types;

Peptic   found in the stomach and gullet, (also known as Gastric Ulcers).

Duodenal   in the top part of the small intestine.

The patient often feels persistently hungry and this is only relieved by the intake of food. Other symptoms include nausea, pain and sickness. These breaks or erosions in the stomach allow the digestive acid to reach the sensitive area underneath, causing the pain and nausea. The presence of blood in the faeces can be a symptom (not to be confused with fresh blood of piles.)

DRUGS FROM CHEMIST

If you suspect you have ulcers you should not treat yourself but see a doctor. If you have persistent indigestion this could be ulcers. Do not make the mistake of constantly taking indigestion remedies to cover the symptoms.

DRUGS FROM DOCTOR

Drug	Information	Possible Side Effects
Antacids: **Milk of Magnesia,** **Actol etc.**	These dilute or neutralise the acid in the stomach. (See Indigestion for a fuller list).	Aluminium drugs may cause constipation.
Mucosal **Strengtheners:** —De No1 —Pyrogostrone —Biogastrone —Bioral Gel —Sucralfate —Antepsin	These help replace the lost mucosa or lining of the stomach.	May cause water retention and should be avoided by old people and those with high blood pressure. May turn faeces black.

ULCERS *(continued)*

DRUGS FROM DOCTOR

Drug	Information	Possible Side Effects
H₂ Antagonists: —Tagamet 　Cimetidine —Ranitidine 　Zantac	These help reduce or stop the production of acid in the stomach. This gives the ulcer chance to heal. May be given for a period of time or indefinitely. Ranitidine clashes and interacts with fewer other drugs.	Cimetidine may interfere with other drugs. Consult a doctor if in doubt. These are a type of anti-histamine drug. (See Antihistamine drugs).
Ardimuscarinics: —Pirenzepine 　Gastrozepin	They block the nerve signal to the cells which make stomach acid.	Constipation and dry mouth.
Misoprostol	Used specifically for NSAID induced ulceration.	Severe diarrhoea. Abdominal pain, flatulance, nausea.

VERRUCAS (See Warts)

VERTIGO (See Dizziness)

VOMITING (See Sickness)

CONSULT YOUR DOCTOR OR PHARMACIST BEFORE TAKING MEDICATION

WARTS

Warts are caused by a virus and are transmissable from person to person. This said, they are not highly contageous (i.e. caught by touch) and if you have a natural immunity to them you will probably not catch them. If you are in any doubt as to whether a mark on the skin is a wart, or anything else come to that, always see your GP to check it out. This is especially true if the wart weeps pus or bleeds.

Treatment for warts is available. However most will go down of their own accord when the body develops an immunity to them. Sometimes liquid nitrogen is used to freeze them, or laser treatment. Genital warts are infectious and should be treated by a doctor.

DRUGS FROM CHEMIST

Drug	Information	Possible Side Effects
Formaldehyde 3% **Formaldehyde 1.5%** —Veracur	Always use the safest preparation possible.	Formaldehyde can have unpredictable results.
Salicylic Acid —Verrugon —Salactol —Duofilm —Cuplex	Most anti-wart preparations work by removing the top layer of skin and then destroying the underlying epidermis.	Can cause severe skin irritation. Avoid unaffected skin.
Glutaraldehyde 10% —Glutarol —Diswart —Verucasep		May irritate and sensitise the skin. Avoid normal skin.
Benzalkonium —Callusolve		Avoid normal skin.
Podophyllin —Posalfilin	Some anti-wart preparations are available from the doctor. These are types of Podophyllin including, Condyline & Warticon.	Do not allow to touch normal skin. Avoid in pregnancy. Do not use on face.

WHOOPING COUGH (See Children's Ailments)